INTERNATIONAL BESTSELLER

A DIFFERENT REALITY

Growing through
our mental health journey together

CHARLIE AND NERISSA TRINDADE

First Edition

Published in 2021

Contact the authors: www.NerissaTrindade.com

ISBN 978-0-6450649-5-7 (Hardcover)
ISBN 978-0-6450649-4-0 (Paperback)
ISBN 978-0-6450649-3-3 (E-book)

Editing by Madhulika Banerjee
Cover design by Rosalyn Ng
Book layout by Marvin Tojos

Our paths may be different, our journeys unique;
while at times it can seem like we have a different
reality, at the end of the day, we're all the same.
We all want to be understood, loved and accepted.

When the going gets tough, the tough get growing.

We dedicate this book to each other, to our family
and friends, to the professionals who guide us
and those who continue to support us.

To those navigating life with a mental health diagnosis and
to all those caring for someone, we hear you, we see you.

Know that you matter, your stories matter.
And that there is always hope.

This book contains discussions of emotional and mental well-being as well as themes of self-harm and suicide that may trigger some readers.

Reader discretion advised.

If you or someone you know needs help, please contact your local mental health care service.

ABOUT THE AUTHORS

Charlie was born and brought up in the United Kingdom and completed her nursing degree in Wales. Having specialised in haematology and oncology, she has decades of extensive experience working in the public, private and voluntary health sectors.

Being a nursing professional and a patient herself, she possesses the incredibly unique perspective that comes from having seen and experienced both sides of the healthcare system. She now draws on her professional qualifications as well as her lived experience of navigating life with both physical and mental health conditions to help inspire and motivate those on similar journeys.

Charlie is passionate about helping others and is working towards opening a foundation to support people who are vulnerable and disadvantaged in their community. She looks forward to incorporating her love for animals into caring for them.

Nerissa was born in India and moved to Australia in her early twenties. She is a professional keynote speaker who has inspired audiences globally and a mindset and transformation coach with years of experience as a change management expert. She is also the bestselling author of her book, *Growing Through*, an autobiographical narrative documenting her own transformation through her coming out journey.

As a migrant, gay woman of colour and a carer for her wife, Charlie, she is no stranger to crisis and adversity. She is known for her positive energy, rational thinking and calm demeanor under extreme pressure.

She is committed to coaching and empowering people to unlock their true potential and thrive both personally and professionally. Nerissa believes in growing through — not going through — life, because anything is possible when you are able to be yourself, believe in yourself and back yourself.

CONTENTS

CHAPTER ONE
THE DIAGNOSIS

I sat at my desk trembling. My computer was broadcasting my thoughts on a large screen to the rest of the team in the office. I was terrified and felt frozen to the spot. I stared at the screen rigid with fear. I could tell they were all watching me. I managed to walk to a quiet room and shut the door and wondered how I could get the chip out of my leg? It was monitoring me and sending out my thoughts to everyone around me. They all knew what I was thinking. There was no escape.

I wrote this in a notebook a few years ago. I was just coming out of a psychotic episode. When I look back at this now, these lines startle me; it almost feels as if they were written by another person. That's because it really is a different reality.

I live with schizoaffective disorder and post-traumatic stress disorder (PTSD). I was first diagnosed with schizoaffective disorder eight years ago, but had been previously treated for PTSD and depression for many years intermittently. Looking back with the knowledge I have now, I am able to recognise symptoms of schizoaffective disorder long before it was first diagnosed. I have battled with my mental health since my early 20s. But it took me a long time to ask for help and go some way to understanding my diagnoses, which led to poor coping behaviours when I was younger. Mental health wasn't as well recognised back in the 80s and 90s and it was hard to find someone I could turn to. I did see one GP (General Practitioner) when I was 22 who started me on antipsychotics, but I didn't know why she prescribed them and was too unwell to ask or understand. I only took the medication for a couple of days and decided to not go back to see her again as I didn't know if I could trust her. A classic example of my paranoia.

The first psychiatrist I saw explained to me that PTSD is a mental health condition that occurs following the experience or threat of a terrifying event. It can be anything — bushfires, war, sexual abuse, or a serious accident. I have experienced symptoms of PTSD to varying degrees for most of my adult life following significant past trauma and continue to do so. For me, symptoms of PTSD include reliving incidents of my past with flashbacks and nightmares, avoiding anything related to what happened back then, and negative changes in my mood and thinking. I feel numb and detached. I also get hyper-alert and feel on edge, as if I'm waiting for something to happen. My PTSD symptoms impact and make the treatment of my schizoaffective disorder more complex and challenging.

So what exactly is schizoaffective disorder? Most people aren't familiar with this diagnosis and it is often poorly understood. My current psychiatrist and I discussed that it is a diagnosis made when someone shows symptoms of schizophrenia (usually psychosis) and a mood disorder — either bipolar disorder or depression. I experience it as the depressive type whereas others may be diagnosed with the bipolar disorder type.

Psychosis indicates that someone has lost contact with reality. Symptoms might include auditory and/or visual hallucinations and/or delusions, which means seeing things that aren't there, hearing voices, or having false beliefs. Some people might also experience alternate forms of hallucinations, for example, olfactory hallucinations.

The specific symptoms of schizoaffective disorder vary between individuals but there is a major mood disorder episode and a two-week psychotic episode which is experienced when the mood component is absent. For me, I struggle with symptoms of depression, such as feelings of worthlessness and sadness. I experience hallucinations where I see people that aren't there and hear voices that are primarily derogatory in nature but turn to commanding when I'm severely unwell. I also experience delusions such as having fixed beliefs about being watched, followed, or monitored. All of this is accompanied by reduced social functioning and communication which, together with the psychotic symptoms and impaired concentration, make it difficult for me to perform basic everyday tasks.

Some people with PTSD, depression and/or schizoaffective disorder experience thoughts and behaviours around deliberate self-harm. This has been true for me since I was nine years old. For me, self-harm was a means to express myself when I couldn't find any other outlet for my emotions. If I was sad, scared, or distressed, this provided a release. As I got older and found different ways to speak my truth, the behaviour stopped. However, the thoughts do still return at times when I'm struggling, but it's something I'm now able to discuss with my wife, Nerissa; my psychotherapist; and my psychiatrist when I need to.

In the past, I have also been suicidal and made attempts on my life. Back then, I actually wanted to end my life. I did not want to live. The pain was too hard to bear and I couldn't see any way out. This is separate from when I used to self-harm to deal with overwhelming emotions but had no intention of killing myself. These days, the suicidal thoughts I have are different. They only manifest when the voices I hear get intense. The voices might tell me to kill myself, and this can put my safety at risk if I act on them, but I myself don't want to die or get injured in any way. I want to live. I'm sure of that now but, I've had these thoughts and feelings for a long time, and it is one of the reasons why I saw my psychotherapist in the first place.

Being able to trust my psychotherapist who encouraged me to see a psychiatrist was an extremely important step for me. I was at a very low point in my life and found myself totally disconnected from my friends and family. I was just about functioning at work while struggling with what I thought was PTSD again. In my distressed state, I couldn't distinguish between being hyper-vigilant and being psychotic. In fact, lack of insight itself is also a feature of psychosis. I was barricading myself into my apartment as soon as I got home from work, trying desperately to contain the voices inside my head.

This is an insight into what I was going through:

I was sitting in the corner of my bedroom in my ground floor apartment in silence. I had barricaded the doors. He was banging at the front door trying to get in. His voice was getting louder telling me he was watching me and there was no escape. He said he was there to take care of me if only I'd let him in. I cried motionless for hours and wondered how many more times he would come back.

Seeing a psychiatrist at this point in my life was a game-changer for me. As a patient, I was irritable, frustrated, withdrawn, and highly paranoid. I found it difficult to explain what was going on inside my head. I was once again diagnosed with PTSD and depression and was started on medications to help. After a few appointments, I decided that I needed to see a female psychiatrist and got a referral. She diagnosed me with schizoaffective disorder after treating me for a couple of years and I was subsequently admitted to a hospital for psychosis.

When I was diagnosed with PTSD and depression, it made sense to me. They were conditions I had heard of and my symptoms clearly fit the assessment criteria. I was also able to read up on them and get some clarity about my mental health. It was a relief more than anything as I was able to finally put a name to what was happening and find the path towards treating it and hopefully feeling better. But being diagnosed with schizoaffective disorder was quite the opposite initially. When my psychiatrist said those words to me, I had mixed emotions. Firstly, I'd never heard of the condition before. I had heard of schizophrenia and mood disorders but not as a condition together. I had preconceived notions about these diagnoses and needed to go a long way before I could understand them fully. Secondly, after listening to my psychiatrist and doing some further reading of my own, I actually got angry with her and went into denial mode. I couldn't believe that I could have a condition that included psychosis. How had I missed it? Was this actually real? But surely all these symptoms could be explained by PTSD? They really couldn't, but it took me a long time to accept that. In fact, denial continues to be a close friend even today.

I needed to see a psychiatrist to confirm my diagnosis of PTSD and depression and later to be diagnosed with schizoaffective disorder. This was significant for me because they are treated in different ways. Part of me still felt anger and resentment about it. I wanted to be 'normal', whatever that is. It didn't seem fair. I'd had enough to deal with in my life so far, and now this? But eventually, there was also some relief. Relief that I could put a name to it, relief I had a level of understanding about it, and relief that I could accept my diagnosis and be treated appropriately. By getting the right diagnosis, I was able to start on the right medication for the right condition, and this really changed my life.

From here on, the goal seemed simple — I had to stay on track, trust my diagnosis, and continue with treatment. However, I would learn in time that living with a mental health diagnosis is actually much more complex than that. It is a layered, challenging, and multi-faceted experience that impacts nearly every aspect of the life of the person who's living with it, and also the lives of their carers and loved ones.

CHAPTER TWO
FINDING OUT

Mental Health? Depression? Psychosis!

These were all alien topics for me. When I was growing up in India in the 1980s, none of this was ever discussed or brought up in conversation. In fact, mental health wasn't even a consideration for most people I knew. The cultural and societal expectation was that everyone should just get up and get on with it. So there was never really an option to not be okay or to say that you were struggling mentally. Mental well-being, as a concept, just didn't seem to exist.

Yes, I had heard of psychiatrists and psychologists even back then. I had this vague concept that the professions existed, but I didn't really know of anyone who went to see them. You'd hear of people going to visit doctors and surgeons, but nobody ever said that they're going to see their therapist for their mental well-being. To be honest, I didn't even know what the difference between a psychiatrist and a psychologist was.

When I look back now, I realise that there must have been people who were struggling with some kind of mental health condition, most of whom were probably never diagnosed. Those people were just written off as 'mad'. I remember there was this older lady in our neighbourhood whom we'd often see across the street, yelling and screaming as if she was terrified of something. No one ever stopped to help her or to try and understand what she was going through. Instead, people just called her crazy and walked on.

As I got older, I'd hear of the occasional person suffering from depression. All anyone would say was, "Oh, they're really sad" or "Oh, they're really withdrawn" and based on that, one would make the assumption that they weren't coping well or were struggling to function and perform day-to-day activities. And that's all I knew of mental health — or didn't know really.

When I moved to Australia, I became more familiar with the concept of stress and anxiety, mostly in the context of balancing work and life commitments. But then again, it wasn't something that came up in everyday conversation. I remember once hearing about a TV show where one of the storylines revolved around a character that had bipolar disorder. My understanding was that people with bipolar disorder experienced extreme changes in their mood and went from feeling extremely happy to extremely sad. Right or wrong, that's all I knew then.

So when I first met Charlie all those years ago, I had no real understanding of what mental health was. We met and became friends and started spending a lot of time together. We really enjoyed each other's company. I found myself drawn to her. We seemed to be able to talk about most things quite comfortably and openly.

As we spent more time together and got to know each other better, Charlie shared with me that she had a mental health diagnosis. She told me about her past trauma and about the PTSD associated with it. My initial reaction was, "Oh, okay. I had absolutely no idea." In all the time that we'd spent together, I hadn't clocked it. I hadn't noticed any of the signs, but then again I wasn't aware of what the symptoms were.

To be very honest, I felt way out of my depth here. I'd never had any actual conversations around mental health with anyone before. So I didn't really know what to say or how to respond. But our friendship had been based on open and honest communication right from the beginning, so I felt comfortable asking her a few questions and allowing her to explain things to me. Back then, I felt she too was still coming to terms with her diagnosis and figuring out what it all meant.

As Charlie and I grew closer, I often contemplated the idea of being in a relationship with her. But Charlie's mental health diagnosis concerned me. I had questions about our future, questions about how our relationship would work if she got unwell. If things didn't work out, would I be able to leave? If I did leave, would she be able to cope? What if she got unwell, would I be able to cope? All valid questions, I guess, when you're considering a new relationship, but her mental health diagnosis added to my hesitation. I wanted to be certain that I could commit to what was needed in the relationship. It took me many months to say yes, to be certain that I was ready to make that commitment. When I look back now though, I realise there was so much that I didn't know. So much that we both didn't know.

For instance, Charlie didn't go through a period of being severely unwell during the time that we were friends. I knew she'd been struggling with PTSD, but back then we weren't living together, so I didn't really know what her day-to-day experience of that was like. I remember she would have days when she needed to shut down and just recharge. And I was comfortable with giving her the time and space she needed. To be honest, I didn't really know what to expect long term. It was this feeling of ambiguity and uncertainty. But the relationship was new and we were happy to take things one day at a time and work through it all together.

Charlie had mentioned to me that she was on psychiatric medication and that she'd been seeing a psychiatrist and psychotherapist regularly. That was when I first began to understand the difference between the two professions. As I understand it, psychiatrists are doctors who specialise in Psychiatry and can prescribe psychiatric medication whereas psychologists and psychotherapists are therapy-based practitioners who help you deal with day-to-day emotions and stress by suggesting strategies and additional therapies to manage the diagnosis and help with everyday functioning.

Eight weeks into our relationship, Charlie had a serious motorbike accident that resulted in severe injuries all down her right side, leading to multiple surgeries and treatments. Understandably, this took a toll on her mental health too. But given the severity of her physical injuries, I feel the mental health aspect initially took a bit of a backseat. In the first few months of our relationship, Charlie didn't experience any mental health breakdowns. Things were hard, there was a lot to get adjusted to. We moved in together. But all things considered, I felt she was doing okay.

It was a few weeks into physical rehab, when Charlie was recovering post-surgery, that I received a call from her one afternoon. She told me she could see foxes coming out of the air vents in her room. Having never been on the receiving end of a call like that, my initial reaction was, "What? What are you seeing?" I thought maybe it was a reaction to one of the pain medications she was on. But on arriving at the hospital and speaking with her and her treating team as well as her therapist, I understood that Charlie was experiencing hallucinations. Her psychiatrist increased one of her medications slightly and after a few days, things were back on an even keel. That was my very first experience of Charlie's hallucinations.

We were about a year into our relationship when Charlie experienced an episode of paranoia for the first time since we'd been together. I remember her being terrified. She was convinced that there was a microchip implanted in her right leg that she felt was monitoring her thoughts and broadcasting them to people from her past. She felt extremely scared and unsafe. I write this now with a much better understanding of Charlie's diagnosis, but back then this was completely new territory for me. I was scared too. I didn't know what to expect, what to say or do. Should I deny what is happening? Should I tell her it isn't true? Should I support her thinking? How best do I help her? I had no clue.

I then remembered having watched an episode on the medical drama series, *Grey's Anatomy*, where a patient with schizophrenia was convinced that the surgeons had placed cameras in his stomach that were monitoring his thoughts. He wouldn't let anyone come near to treat him. One of the doctors then brought in his scans and showed him that there were, in fact, no cameras inside him. She then left the scans in his room so he could look at them and feel reassured whenever those thoughts returned.

I thought, why not try the same? I took out one of the old X-ray films of Charlie's leg from after the accident and showed it to her. She was able to see that there were no chips there and that reassured her. However, the thoughts did return and once again, it took a tweaking of medications, multiple therapy sessions, as well as shutting down from the world outside, for Charlie to come through that episode without requiring hospitalisation.

That was the first time I witnessed what Charlie was going through. It was, understandably, challenging and scary for both of us in different ways. After these episodes, Charlie's psychiatrist diagnosed her with schizoaffective disorder. This is a rarer diagnosis than schizophrenia. The way I have come to understand schizoaffective disorder is as a combination of psychosis along with a mood disorder. For Charlie, it is psychosis and depression, and in many ways, it creates a different reality for her.

It took the both of us some time to wrap our heads around the new diagnosis but looking back now, I think it was particularly hard for Charlie. I feel it takes a while for anyone to understand and come to terms with a particular diagnosis, and for some people with schizoaffective disorder, fighting the diagnosis itself can be a feature of the condition, which, of course, then makes coming to terms with it even harder.

For me, this was all brand new territory. I was just starting to learn what all of this meant and was trying to grapple with what this would mean for our future. Irrespective of what the final diagnosis was, I knew we'd still have a battle on our hands. We'd still have to figure out how to live with this diagnosis.

I feel getting the right diagnosis helped Charlie better understand her condition and what it meant for her on a day-to-day basis. It also helped her treating team come up with the best treatment plan to manage the diagnosis. And it helped me, as her carer, to access more information and gain a better understanding of how I can best help her.

Over the years, I've been able to come to terms with what this means for us, for our relationship and the life we're journeying through together. I now have a much better understanding of her triggers, medications and treatment plans. This has enabled us to build a life that doesn't revolve around her diagnosis but continues to evolve and thrive knowing that this is ongoing for us.

CHAPTER THREE
LIVED EXPERIENCE

Living with schizoaffective disorder and PTSD can be extremely lonely, isolating, and confronting. It sure has its challenges. A lot of what I experience is hidden. It can be a very dark world to enter into. I tell the people closest to me most of what goes on inside my head but it's generally only after the fact that I am able to cope with telling them what's been happening. Often this communication is via text or email with Nerissa, even if she's only sitting in the next room. Establishing these modes of contact when I'm unwell has been crucial for us, particularly when I'm feeling unsafe and am unable to express it.

My mental health is unpredictable, uncertain, and influences most parts of our lives. I go through periods when I'm well and feel good about myself. On days like these, I have a great connection with Nerissa; we are able to really laugh together and enjoy each other's company. We feel close and safe in a deeply loving relationship. On an average day, I wake up in the morning feeling energised after a good night's sleep. I shower and make plans for the day. This could involve taking our dog for a walk or catching up with a friend for a coffee. I enjoy having lunch with Nerissa when she's home and sometimes spend the afternoon with a support worker who I have over three times a week. We might head out to run errands or go grocery shopping. A day like this is refreshing. It helps me recharge my batteries and enjoy some of the simple things in life.

Sometimes even doing these basic things can trigger a relapse. The supermarket can be an overwhelming place when I'm hearing voices or having paranoid thoughts, which is most of the time, even when I'm well. What marks a good day from a bad one is the difference in the intensity of these voices and the kind of things I hear them saying. This is not like listening to music for me; it's more like being cornered by a gang of people with all of them talking and shouting at me at the same time. In the supermarket, there are customers chatting, staff talking, kids screaming and loud announcements being made. All while I'm trying to read a shopping list and select the items I'm buying. This might not sound difficult until the voices kick in, saying: *I'm watching you, I'm following you, I'm never far behind you, you can't do anything for yourself*.

The voices I hear as part of schizoaffective disorder are known as auditory hallucinations. They happen inside my head and no one else can hear them. They are extremely distressing and interrupt connection with everyone around me, including Nerissa. They are an isolating experience and vary at different times. For the most part, I largely hear two male voices that are known to me, or sometimes just one of them. At other times, I hear a third separate voice that I perceive to be the voice of God. On the good days, the voices are derogatory in nature and I've learnt to flick them off and take back control of my mind.

Then there's a relapse which always leads to a bad day. I wake up in the morning feeling exhausted after a night full of PTSD-related nightmares which I usually only remember in snippets. Then I have a visual hallucination of my abuser standing at the end of my bed. I'm terrified and want to shout out but I'm too scared. I turn to Nerissa for reassurance but I can't speak up to tell her what I see. Breathe Charlie, breathe, I tell myself. I turn back and, thank goodness, he's gone. I get out of bed in trepidation. I wonder what awaits me. The voices are intense.

You're pathetic, you're useless, you have a chip in your leg monitoring your thoughts, you deserve everything that comes your way. If you don't jump in front of a train today I'll kill you. I'm monitoring your thoughts and can broadcast them at my will. If you talk to anyone about this I'll rape you again.

My anxiety flares up which then triggers a PTSD flashback to my trauma. I feel I'm being attacked from all angles. I'm hypervigilant. I remain in a state of alertness as I try to manage these experiences of PTSD alongside schizoaffective disorder.

My bad day continues. The day has only begun but I already feel so exhausted. The voices aren't letting up. I have some breakfast and head back to bed. I know the nightmares will go on but sleep is the only thing I can think about. I explain to Nerissa that it's a bad day but I haven't got the energy to explain why, and anyway I'm too terrified to talk because of the voices. Once in bed, he's there again. There is no escaping it. I hide under the duvet and hope there will be a reprieve. I fall asleep briefly and wake up startled with a nightmare. The voices have shifted up a gear. They're now constant. He's going to harm me or worse unless I do as he says. They're saying the same thing over and over again. It's like a running commentary. Two voices talking at the same time. Talking to each other about me. They threaten me. Tell me to hurt myself. It's overwhelming. The voices keep changing. They get louder and more frequent. Their intensity increases and they continuously tell me to hurt myself or they'll kill me. I can't put into words the level of fear and terror I experience. I know I have to do something to shut them up.

Nerissa.

I send her a text explaining what's happening. I can't speak. She comes into the room and instantly there is a shift as 'he' goes away. I can't see him anymore. She tells me I'm safe. It's okay. She's with me. I cry. Actually, I sob. I've frightened myself that I might have actually acted on the voices. There are also delusions accompanying the voices. False paranoid beliefs that I'm being watched, that my abusers are never far behind me, that I have a chip in my leg that is transmitting and broadcasting my thoughts again to other people. I think that I can't take any medication or I'm going to be killed. I feel terribly distraught, but at least I have found some way to convey my thoughts and feelings to Nerissa.

Luckily, I have my regular appointment with my psychotherapist scheduled for that afternoon. I discuss it with Nerissa. We agree that she will come with me and in the meantime, I will take some medication to ease what I'm experiencing and try to sleep again. I rest in bed with her there and fall asleep. What a relief. Nerissa wakes me up before lunch and gives me something to eat. The intensity of the voices and delusions have reduced a little. We head to the appointment. Once I'm there, I feel safer. I show my psychotherapist the text I sent to Nerissa so that she knows where I'm up to. She acknowledges my distress and supports me while we talk it through. I think I know what's coming next. She's concerned about my safety and says I need to be in hospital. I resist initially but I soon realise I don't have the energy to fight this one. She reassures me that it'll only be for a few days so that

I can shut down. Nerissa agrees and we leave with a plan to go to the hospital.

This kind of relapse can be triggered by something like anxiety, or by nothing at all. It can be rapid or slow. It can involve a hospital admission or not. In 2020, I had five hospital admissions. Other years, I've had one or two. These days the admissions are shorter, up to a week. However, if I require medication changes, that often leads to longer admissions. The shorter admissions are designed to keep me safe and let the intense period of voices and delusions pass without causing me harm. I describe it as a computer rebooting. My mind becomes overloaded and needs to shut down so that the reboot process can begin.

When I have a relapse, it often starts with anxiety and with a pattern of thinking and behaviour that includes denial. Denying I have a mental health condition is a big part of living with it. I question the diagnosis and also question whether I need medication. I read a lot about schizoaffective disorder and try to find a get-out clause. A different way to explain my condition. Then, I proclaim that I don't need the medication even though it has given me the biggest relief from my symptoms. Instead, I believe my condition has been caused by my medication. I argue the toss with my therapist and Nerissa. I tell them I don't need it, there are too many side effects. I tell them there are other ways to treat mental health. That my psychiatrist is plotting against me. Then my emotional and mental state deteriorates. The voices in my head really crank up. They change from being derogatory to commanding. *Don't take medication. Take an overdose of medication. Jump in front of a train. Jump out of a window. Don't talk to anyone, not even Nerissa.* On the background runs a constant commentary of — *If you tell someone, they'll lock you up.*

Below is an excerpt from an email I sent to my psychotherapist after one such experience. It's interesting that the voice is telling me that I can't tell anyone and yet I'm emailing my therapist. It shows my struggle and confusion but also how much I trust her.

He was telling me to stop taking my medication. He said I'm not unwell. It's all in me. It's my fault. I have to stop the meds and I can't tell anyone or he'll rape me again. I tried to challenge the voices. Fight back. But he got louder and louder. I couldn't hear myself think. I had to do as he said.

A couple of years back, it took three days of not taking medication for me to tell Nerissa. She remained calm, and focused on what was needed to get me back on track. It took a hard conversation for her to be able to persuade me to go into hospital. When I'm unwell, I generally believe that I don't need to go in which makes it difficult for Nerissa and my therapist who are usually involved in getting an admission organised. I still fight it, which is perplexing to me when I'm well. This is an excerpt from another email I sent to my therapist that provides an insight into how I feel in these times:

I need to set some boundaries around our conversation today. Please don't ask me anything about being watched or listened to. They are at work. The doctors are plotting against me and 'he' keeps coming down from the vent in the ceiling and standing at the end of my bed. We went home [from hospital] *for the afternoon on Sunday which was lovely except for the cameras in the apartment block. Did I draw you a map showing you where they were? There were nine. Yesterday we had a group session* [in therapy] *on thought monitoring. The group was monitoring my thoughts. I will be talking to the doctor and asking why I have to be on this medication. I really don't think I need it. Can you agree with me on this?*

It took a long time and a lot of trial and error to arrive at the medication regimen that can help me cope with these thoughts and voices. I currently take an antidepressant, a mood stabilizer, and antipsychotics. I went through multiple drugs and different doses to get to a point where I could function, albeit with sporadic hospital admissions. In order to keep my outpatient and inpatient psychiatrists on the same page, I have a Safety Plan in place, the template for which you can find at the end of this book. The Safety Plan exists to ensure that my care can be streamlined regardless of whether I am at home or in hospital. When I go into hospital to shut down, I usually need my long-term medications to stay the same while I take additional medication to help me deal with my acute symptoms. The Safety Plan is kept updated in my hospital file, so whoever takes over my care knows where we're at. This can be a huge asset when different psychiatrists treat you in the community and at the hospital.

The other people who have been involved in writing my Safety Plan are Nerissa and my psychotherapist. Nerissa and I came up with a 1-10 scale that we felt would help the both of us gain a better understanding of how I'm doing. We use this scale to determine my voices score and a suicide score, with one being low and 10 being high. We both felt that expressing myself through this scale could help me in my communication with Nerissa, and with the professionals involved in my care. After creating the scale, we agreed to implement it via a daily check-in and it's really helped us both.

As you can see, living with a mental health diagnosis is complex. My diagnosis comes with many varied and interrelated symptoms. Nerissa is happy to support me throughout my journey but we understand that I need to see a psychotherapist and psychiatrist so that the professionals involved in my care can support us both. There can be many different people and factors to consider. I'm lucky because I have incredible support from Nerissa, friends, family, and professionals. However, this hasn't happened overnight. It takes time to build a strong support network but this is totally worth the time and effort.

CHAPTER FOUR
CARER'S JOURNEY

"You are safe. I promise, you are safe."

I've found myself saying these three words to my wife on numerous occasions. These are words I've often repeated to myself too — she is safe.

Yes, I am a carer. It is a role I now have, one of the many that I fulfil on a daily basis. But, what is a carer, really? In a general sense, a carer is anyone who provides care for someone else. Parents are carers; sometimes, children are carers for their parents. At times, we may care for a partner or a loved one, a friend, or someone in our community.

When I explore my carer journey in this chapter, I refer specifically to my role as a mental health carer for Charlie. Even though Charlie also lives with a physical disability that we'll address in the next chapter, my focus here is on what it means to care for someone living with a mental health condition.

Often, becoming a carer isn't a choice. It's a role we find ourselves in based on the nature of our relationship with the person who needs to be cared for. I did know Charlie was living with a mental health condition when we first met, but I didn't necessarily know how that would play out in our lives, and the role I would find myself in. All I knew was that I was in love with her and I was willing to do whatever it took.

For a long time, I didn't even consider myself to be a carer. I simply saw it as part of my role as a partner, and I didn't quite understand the physical, emotional and mental toll it was taking on me. It was only when I acknowledged my role as a carer that I was able to get the help I needed, which then allowed me to better care for myself and Charlie.

Living with someone with a mental health condition can be extremely challenging. You might often find yourself experiencing a range of mixed emotions. Over the years, I've felt angry, frustrated, scared, uncertain, and often very alone. I've also experienced loss and grief. But with this comes deep love, care, concern, respect and empathy for my wife. Understanding what Charlie has to navigate on a day-to-day basis has enabled me to experience and process my own emotions without letting them adversely impact our relationship.

The nature of being a mental health carer is often cyclic. It can feel like you're on an endlessly looping rollercoaster where you go from having a really good day to having a particularly bad one. As Charlie mentions, it's a cycle of hospital admissions, therapy sessions, medication and treatment plans, coupled with relapses of psychosis and paranoia, all of which can start to form a pattern over a period of time. Even for the carer, this can feel relentless with no real break or way out. However, understanding the cyclic nature of the illness and its patterns has allowed me, after much trial and error, to learn to live with the uncertainty.

On a good day, Charlie and I have a beautiful relationship built on love, trust, respect, open and honest communication, humour, and a lot of fun. We got married in 2017, and have been together for a long time now. We share a lovely home together, with our little dog, and have built a life that works for us. A life that gives us immense joy, pleasure, happiness and fulfilment. A life surrounded by friends who care and family that support us no matter what. On a good day, life is good and there isn't really anything we can complain about.

But as you can imagine, on a bad day, life looks significantly different. On such days, especially when the voices are commanding and their intensity and frequency increase, one phone call and a few seconds can change everything. There have been times when I've been at work and received an SOS phone call from Charlie, not knowing whether that's the last call I'll ever receive. *When I get home, will she still be alive?*

I recall an instance when Charlie was in hospital as the voices had become really intense and commanding in nature. I was at work when Charlie called and told me that the louder voice was demanding that she jump in front of a train or she would be killed. I immediately called the hospital to let them know and then started to make my way there. The quickest route was by train. I was sitting on the train when it suddenly halted midway. I assumed it was a technical fault or another train passing, but then the guard announced that the train had been halted because there'd been a fatality. Someone had jumped onto the tracks.

Instantly, my heart sank. Our last phone conversation was playing repeatedly in my head. I pulled out my phone and tried to ring

Charlie. No response. I was terrified. I knew she was in hospital and could not have made it to the station, but I couldn't dismiss the thought either. *Could it be her?*

I hate to admit it, but this is the reality I live with. I know she won't do anything, I have to believe that. I know she doesn't want to, but what if one day it gets too much?

It can be extremely frightening for carers to live with these feelings. It is also enormously challenging to navigate this level of uncertainty and fear on a regular basis. It took me a long time to acknowledge my feelings and recognise what it means to constantly live without knowing what the next day, month or year will look like. All of a sudden, I found myself living with a certain level of anxiety that I had never necessarily been diagnosed with. As someone who generally likes to be in control of their situation and surroundings, it was difficult for me to accept that I would now have to journey through life with this extreme level of uncertainty.

I'm also a person of logic and reason and pride myself on rational thinking. Yet, when dealing with mental health, no form of logic or reason ever wins. Once the paranoia sets in, all logic and reason go out the window. While this can be extremely scary and challenging for the carer, it is even more distressing for the person experiencing it. As Charlie describes it, everything that she experiences, everything that she hears or sees, feels real. No amount of logic or reasoning can help, because, for the person experiencing it, it is very much their reality. It's just a different reality. So instead of denying her feelings, what helps is for me to acknowledge that this is, in fact, what she is experiencing and to let her know that in my reality, she is safe and secure.

Often, being a carer also means having to make some hard decisions. One of the symptoms of psychosis is not having insight into being unwell. So Charlie often does not realise or necessarily believe that she's becoming unwell, which means I, as her carer, have to step in and play bad cop. Telling the person you love that they aren't well is hard enough, but ensuring that they stick to medication and treatment plans is often even harder.

At first, the symptom of not wanting to take medication would really frustrate me. To the average person it seems perfectly logical — if you're unwell and there is medication available that can help, why wouldn't you take it? But here too, I slowly grew to understand the different reality that Charlie experiences, how things look from her perspective when she's unwell. I now get that taking medication you think is potentially poisoning you can seem terrifying, and I've learnt how to work around this with her.

Initially, hospital admissions would frighten me too. The early hospital admissions were very different to the ones we now experience. They were usually much longer, sometimes stretching up to two months, and often involved medication changes. I remember one such hospital admission where a number of medications had been tried and tested, and as each one got eliminated, our list of viable options kept reducing. Nothing seemed to be working. Finally, after several weeks, one drug proved to be effective. However, this drug required really close monitoring as it had severe side effects. Just as we were starting to see some signs of improvement, I remember getting a call from the hospital saying Charlie was having severe chest pain and trouble breathing. I rushed out of work praying all the way that she'd be okay. What had started as an admission to the psych hospital now led to her being rushed to emergency for a potentially life-threatening heart condition. We were lucky that they were able to detect this in time and take her off the drug, but Charlie still had to spend a week in the cardiac unit. While we were relieved her heart was okay, it also meant that we were once again back to the drawing board on what medication could now be trialled. Medication changes in Charlie's case have been quite constant and we understand that this is something we will continue to have to work through.

The purpose of the hospital admissions has slowly shifted over the years. Now they're more of an early intervention for safety, and might involve the occasional medication change. Still, each time Charlie is unwell and the question of a hospital admission is raised, she often says no in the first instance. And in those moments, I'm left with having to make the hard decision of recommending that she be admitted to hospital for her own safety. And each time, once she starts to feel better shortly after being in, she's reassured that it was the right decision. She'll often thank me later, but at that moment, she really isn't pleased with me. But I've learnt now that, in some instances, it's the best decision I can make for her.

Over the years, Charlie has become better at understanding her triggers and symptoms and is sometimes able to indicate to me when she's becoming unwell. I too now know all her triggers and can almost preempt a relapse. I remember Charlie once said she was sorry for ending up in hospital again, to which I responded, "You don't need to be sorry at all, I'm so proud of you for being able to let me know you're struggling and you need help." I often say this, and it might sound a bit morbid, but it's true, "I'd much rather go to a hospital than a morgue."

This is what a relapse can sometimes look like. And, this would often happen while I was working full-time. There have been several instances where I've been on a call with her at work, talking to her and calming her down, and I've then had to go straight into a meeting or deliver a presentation right after. It isn't easy. Having to shift from a personal life crisis and into a professional headspace can be extremely hard. People often talk about work-life balance, but that has never really been a thing for me. For me, it's all part of life and it revolves and merges into one. It is more about understanding priorities and what's important, and for me, Charlie is my top priority every single time.

Being a carer has also had an impact on the types of roles I could apply for and the jobs I've been able to accept throughout my career. With each role, I've found it best to be upfront about what my life looks like. Having flexibility at work has always been crucial for me. It's important for me that the team and the organisation understand my commitments. That being said, I've been a high performer in all my roles whilst being a carer. I attribute a lot of that to the flexible working arrangements at the organisations I've been lucky to work with, as well as the support systems we've built around us. Now that I run my own business, we have even more flexibility and freedom to live life on our own terms, and we've noticed that it's really helped us both.

Being a long-term carer also impacts you physically and emotionally. For example, having Charlie in hospital might seem like a reprieve but some admissions have really taken their toll on me. At first, I found myself trying to manage and control everything – home, work, Charlie's needs in hospital, as well as constant communication with the doctors and her treating team. Needless to say, that got really stressful and overwhelming for me. Over the years, we've found and built support systems that have helped take the load off me, both when she's in hospital as well as at home.

A carer's journey can often be quite an isolating one as not many people understand what you go through on a day-to-day basis. Also, with Charlie being in hospital from time to time, life can sometimes get very lonely. Moreover, topics around suicide, self-harm, psychosis etc., don't really come up in everyday conversation with friends over drinks. So it's crucial that carers have a safe place to share their feelings and get the support they need. I'll share with you in the chapters ahead what support has helped me and enabled me to care better for Charlie.

It's so important that as carers, we understand that we need to be cared for too and that it's okay to ask for help. We need to ensure that we're caring for ourselves, and we've got other people in our corner that are caring for us, so we, in turn, can better care for the people that we love. Having these supports in place has immensely helped me at times when Charlie is severely unwell. If she's suicidal at any time, we know what to do, who to contact, and exactly what steps need to be followed to keep her safe.

This can seem really raw and hard-hitting, but it is essential. These conversations around life and death, the moments where I've come close to losing her, have really put everything else about life and our relationship into perspective. It's what ensures that we never take life or a single day for granted. We know how lucky we are to still be here, to still be together and it's what drives us to keep growing, to keep learning on this journey.

CHAPTER FIVE
PHYSICAL AND MENTAL HEALTH

Up until nine years ago, my general physical health was good. I worked four days a week as a Registered Nurse (RN) in Haematology and Oncology and any time I took off as sick leave was mostly due to my mental health.

Then, I had a motorcycle accident.

I was on my way home from an evening shift at work. It was a cool winter's evening on a Sunday and the roads were pretty clear. I was driving at the speed limit — 50km/hr — when suddenly a car coming from the opposite direction sharply turned right straight in front of me. I had absolutely no chance of avoiding the car and was T-boned and thrown off my motorbike onto the side road. As I hit the tarmac, I felt an excruciating pain in my right leg. I heard someone running towards me and then crouching down beside me. They touched my back and I screamed out in pain, asking them to get their hands off and not touch any part of my body. As an RN, I knew the importance of being assessed by the paramedics before making any movements. By now two other people had come by. I could hear one saying to the other that my leg looked deformed. I had no idea how bad it was, which was probably a good thing at that point. After what felt like an eternity, the ambulance arrived and I heard the reassuring voice of a paramedic telling me they were going to give me something for the pain. "Morphine!" I shouted, knowing nothing else would work. I was freezing cold by now and desperate to get inside the ambulance.

When I came around again, I was in Emergency. I don't recall any of what happened after the paramedics gave me the morphine. I just remember waking up feeling a whole lot warmer and in less pain. I was with it enough to ask a nurse for my phone so I could contact Nerissa.

***

While my understanding of Charlie's mental health had grown gradually over a period of time through our many conversations, the accident came as a complete shock.

We had only been together for about eight weeks. We were still in the initial, early stages of our relationship. We'd normally speak over the phone when Charlie got home after her evening shift; only that night I kept waiting but there was no phone call. I remember calling her flatmate to check if she'd arrived home and whether her phone had died or something, but Charlie's flatmate hadn't heard from her either.

It was getting pretty late and I was now worried. I was just about to leave home to drive to her work when I got a phone call from the Emergency Department, letting me know she'd had an accident. I remember speaking to her and feeling so relieved that she was alive. I rushed to the hospital and found out she'd suffered multiple injuries all down her right side.

***

I was covered in blankets and was in a neck brace when Nerissa arrived. They were about to take me for a CT scan to check if I had any brain or spinal injuries. Thankfully, it came back clear. However, I had sustained multiple injuries all down my right side — a fractured elbow that required reconstruction, and fractures to my femur, tibia, fibular, and toes, all of which necessitated extensive orthopaedic surgery. I also had large degloving injuries to my right lower leg and foot that required debriding and skin grafting by a plastic surgeon.

***

That night, neither of us could've guessed the extent of the impact the accident would have on the rest of our lives. Those few seconds, and someone else's reckless driving, had changed our lives forever.

I didn't really know it then, but from that day, I became Charlie's carer for her physical health too. And since then, the journey has been long and it's been gruelling. It's tested us in ways we never imagined, but it has also taught us a lot.

***

Fast forward four years to 2016. I had already undergone 22 surgeries and had experienced intense acute and chronic pain while my surgeons attempted to save my leg. Each surgery gave us new hope that things would improve, but we were knocked back time after time. It was then that I said enough is enough. I began to consider the possibility of a right below-knee amputation with my surgeon. Within weeks, I was booked in to have the surgery that gave me the ultimate hope that our future could finally change, and this time, our instincts were right. It was one of the best decisions we have made about my physical health treatment.

Since my amputation, I've had surgery on my left wrist after falling and also two spinal surgeries to my lower back for slipped discs. Understandably, my mental health came on this rollercoaster with us and I had many hospital admissions for psychiatric care alongside the admissions for my physical health.

Every surgery I've had has had an impact on my mental health, either at the time itself or further down the track. Anaesthetics themselves are known to have side effects on some people who may experience problems including hallucinations, depression, and psychosis. Couple this with PTSD and schizoaffective disorder, and it is not surprising that I've had relapses and spent so much time in psychiatric hospitals. Physical and mental health are deeply intertwined. When I see my outpatient psychiatrist, she always asks if I'm having any physical health complaints such as pain that may be affecting my mental health. It is an integral part of the assessment.

For me, pain can sometimes be a trigger for episodes of depression and psychosis. The amputation was a life-changing experience and I would never regret it. However, wearing a prosthetic leg comes with its own challenges. I experience changes in the fitting of the leg which causes pain when I mobilise and I feel pain when I have alterations to the prosthetic leg or change to a new prosthetic. I also get phantom limb pain at night on a regular basis which at times impacts my sleep.

While my physical health does have an impact on my mental health, the reverse is also true. My mental health also often influences my physical health. For example, my medication can sometimes lead to dietary changes such as increased appetite or changes in weight, which in turn, affect the fit of my prosthetic leg. This can cause an increase in pain and a lack of motivation to exercise. Further, my problems with taking medication due to psychosis can lead to a range of mental health and physiological symptoms.

What's interesting about being someone with physical and mental health problems is observing the difference in the responses of the people around me. Being an amputee with lived experience of PTSD and schizoaffective disorder gives me a unique perspective on this. With Nerissa, we're in it together regardless of whether it's physical or mental health. Through our relationship, I've learnt to be more open and honest with myself and others regardless of what we're dealing with. I've had to challenge my own internal shame around mental health and accept that we're still learning every day, whether it's about my health or our relationship.

***

Supporting Charlie through the multiple surgeries and caring for her physical needs hasn't been easy. Neither of us has immediate family here with us in Australia, which means I've had to carry the bulk of the responsibility as her sole carer. Whether that's involved making big decisions or being present for every surgery and recovery process, we've been through it all together. The ups and downs have been challenging, and although the physical aspects of this journey have been absolutely gruelling, it doesn't even come close to how difficult the mental health aspect has been.

Charlie's physical disabilities have brought their own challenges, such as pain and learning to live life as an amputee. But the real work has been the constant mental battle of picking her up emotionally after surgeries didn't work or dealing with the lack of confidence the physical injuries brought, in addition to her anxiety and other mental health conditions.

There have been moments after her surgeries where I've stood by Charlie's hospital bed counting every breath to check if she was still breathing. Following one of the early surgeries, I remember her respiratory rate dropped really low and she needed close monitoring. That was scary, extremely scary, but still, nothing compared to how terrified I've been with regard to her mental health, with her suicidal or self-harm thoughts, for example. In some ways, I feel that with the physical aspect, I can see and know what's happening. Even if I can't feel her pain, I can see the injuries and somehow fathom what she must be going through. But with mental health, because it's something that isn't visible, I used to find it extremely hard to understand what Charlie was experiencing, especially when she struggled to articulate herself in any spoken or written form. It's taken us years to work out how to better communicate about her mental health, and that's been such a blessing for both of us individually, and for our relationship.

***

When it comes to my physical health, I have no issues discussing my amputation with most people. But when it comes to my mental health, it's very different on both sides. I never know how much is okay to say. If you talk about being psychotic or having suicidal ideations caused by the voices, many people don't know how to respond. I try to be as lighthearted as possible but none of this really makes for lighthearted conversation.

I was born and brought up in the United Kingdom, where most people traditionally have a 'stiff upper lip' attitude. Meaning we really should just get on with whatever we're dealt with. The first time I was mentally unwell was in my early 20s. I spent five months in hospital over two admissions. My family visited most days which was very supportive. As far as I can recall, we rarely talked about why I was in hospital. That was too difficult a topic for conversation. Most of my friends during this time struggled with visiting. I had two friends who came to visit and discussed how I was feeling but this really wasn't the norm. People are sometimes frightened by mental health. They don't know what to say because they're concerned they'll make the situation worse. So instead, they don't say anything.

Within a week of my motorcycle accident, however, a group of friends from the hospital where I worked came to visit me. There were about ten of them. We laughed and joked as only nurses can about my predicament of being in a plaster cast right from my shoulder down to my toes, and discussed everything in between. They had a great energy and gave me a real boost before being directed away from my room to keep the noise down. Now, I had worked with this group of nurses for two years and had a great rapport with them. We all worked in a highly stressful environment and had each others' backs. It was a lovely team to be part of. However, during those two years, I had had psychiatric admissions to hospital and had found it difficult to keep up my performance at work. But I had not told anyone about my mental health. My manager knew for practical reasons because I needed time off, but it was never discussed. When I'd come back to work after being away, nobody ever asked why I'd been off, it just wasn't mentioned. Perhaps they knew and thought it was better coming from me. I don't know. Shouldn't there be a world where we can talk about our physical and mental health at work equally and openly?

Families too can sometimes struggle with mental health and caring for their loved ones. Members of my family visited during my initial psychiatric hospital admission in Australia and also when I had my accident. Because we're generally more comfortable discussing my physical health, I felt it was much easier and more comfortable for them to support me regarding my accident than during my mental health admissions. However, over the years I've realised that it's good for me to be more open and honest with my family and friends about my mental health. My family now knows about my diagnosis and we're more open in sharing how this plays out.

***

I too struggled with talking about Charlie's mental health at first, particularly with my colleagues and friends at work. Because the accident happened so early in our relationship, the focus was mostly on her physical health. Back then, I too was coming to terms with everything and had a very limited understanding of mental health. I didn't know how to approach the topic, what to share, what not to share. So often it was just easier to focus on the physical aspects rather than on mental health.

However, as time progressed and we started getting our heads around what was happening, I guess we felt easier talking to each other about it. Our understanding and awareness grew and slowly we realised that if we didn't talk about it ourselves, then we were in some way contributing to the stigma associated with mental health. If we couldn't be comfortable talking about it, then how could we expect others to do so? So we decided to start speaking up — with family, friends and colleagues. It's also one of the reasons we wanted to write this book, to share our story, so it helps to create awareness, further the conversation, and break the stigma associated with mental health.

I'm extremely lucky that I've been able to talk about this openly with my mum and sister. Even though mental health was never really discussed in India when I was growing up, things have come a long way since then. My mum and sister have always been really open to discussing hospital admissions, medication changes, and have been involved in all that we've been through over the years. They ask questions, and at times, we all learn together. Having family that I can share all of this with and communicate some really deep and dark stuff to has been extremely helpful. I feel really well-supported, even though they're not here in person. My mum has come and stayed with us for periods of time when Charlie has been very unwell and this has been such a blessing and help for us both.

Our journey to this point has been a complex and complicated process and we've both been through the wringer in terms of physical and mental health complexities.

Over the years, it's been interesting to see the difference in people's reactions, the changes in the way we've coped and communicated about physical and mental health, and also the interrelated impact they've had on our lives.

What we've found is that once we're able to share our personal stories and journeys, both physical and mental health-related, people too are more willing to have conversations and share their own experiences with us.

CHAPTER SIX
TREATMENTS AND OUR EXPERIENCES

In this chapter, we'll share with you our personal experiences of the different mental health treatments that Charlie has tried over the years. We'll outline what's worked, what hasn't, and how some of these continue to help us today.

Know that depending on the diagnosis, treatments can be different and it's best to work with your treating team or that of your loved one to determine the right treatment plan.

PSYCHOTHERAPY

Psychotherapists are therapy-based practitioners who use in-depth psychological approaches to treat people with mental health conditions or help those who might like some support around their general well-being. They work to improve functioning, increase life skills, and change behaviours that can be detrimental to their clients' physical and mental health. They can work with individuals, couples, families or groups. My psychotherapist works systemically with me and involves Nerissa in some sessions.

I have been seeing my current psychotherapist for the past 11 years. I see her once a week when I'm stable and twice a week when I'm unwell. She has supported me through my highs and many lows. When I first started seeing her, I was self-harming and was at one of the lowest points in my life. For months on end, I would go to see her and barely speak at all. I was depressed and psychotic and didn't have the words or the insight to express what was going on. Looking back, I can see it was a safe space for me to just be, which I needed more than anything at the time. She persuaded me to see a psychiatrist in order to consider medication, which I did in time. Shortly afterwards, I became suicidal and attempted to commit suicide with a medication overdose. I ended up as an inpatient in a mental health unit after being treated in Emergency. I spent many weeks there. During this time, I continued my sessions with my psychotherapist over the phone. This was crucial as it provided the continuity I needed and gave me someone to talk to who could really understand what I was going through and offer me the best support. She made me feel safe when nothing else around me seemed safe. I could be exactly as I felt and it was okay. She listened to me regardless of how bizarre I was sounding and accepted me for who I am.

What I get from my sessions with my psychotherapist is unconditional positive regard. She has always got my back, whether I'm well or paranoid. She helps me make sense of my world which can be an extremely scary place and supports me to get the right kind of help when I need it. I can say anything to her and she isn't shocked and doesn't dismiss me. Nothing's off-limits with her. She uses many different approaches to support me and each of them has its own benefits.

***

When Charlie first mentioned to me that she was seeing a psychotherapist regularly, I was really pleased that she was getting the support she needed. Initially, I thought therapy was just her thing. I was like, "Okay, you go off to therapy, sort it out and we'll be fine."

But over the years, I've realised how important it is for me to be heard as well. For me to be able to share my feelings, my concerns, and my own triggers, and be able to independently talk to someone who knows what we're both experiencing.

I see the same psychotherapist Charlie goes to and have really benefited from having individual therapy sessions with her. We've also had many couple sessions over the years to help us navigate some extremely tricky situations. I've found these sessions absolutely invaluable as they have helped me comprehend what Charlie is experiencing and get better at working through things together.

We're now at a place where we have a really good three-way understanding. Charlie speaks to her therapist for approximately one to two hours a week, so there are often instances when I notice some of Charlie's triggers or pick up worsening symptoms outside of her therapy sessions. I relay this to Charlie's therapist so she can better support her; we also organise additional sessions as needed. In the same way, the therapist might sometimes pick up on something during a session that is important for me to know so I can better support Charlie at home, and she relays this back, either through Charlie or via email. I feel there's an immense level of trust and respect that has been built over the years and this has been fundamental to our well-being and our journey of progress. We've both realised that therapy isn't only crisis management but something that can benefit people on a regular and ongoing basis.

PSYCHIATRY

A psychiatrist is a doctor who specialises in diagnosing and treating people with mental health conditions. They prescribe medication for their patients and might provide treatments such as Electroconvulsive Therapy (ECT) or Transcranial Magnetic Stimulation (TMS).

I've been seeing my current psychiatrist for 10 years now. I see her once every four to six weeks when I'm well and once or twice a fortnight when I'm unstable. She manages my overall care and treatment and prescribes any changes in my medication. She works with other psychiatrists at the hospital when I'm admitted there and has been actively involved in developing my Safety Plan. It has been helpful to have her consistently as my needs have changed and evolved over the years. Having one person who has a history of my conditions, medications, and treatments has been invaluable rather than switching between psychiatrists and having to start from scratch each time. My psychiatrist knows me really well by now, which means when I relapse, I don't have to explain too much for her to understand where I'm at. She also liaises with my psychotherapist at times and they work together to support us.

***

When I met Charlie initially, she was already connected with her current psychiatrist. Remember that back then, I didn't even know what the difference was between a psychiatrist and a psychotherapist. I do understand the difference now and I've seen how the two really complement each other when it comes to contributing to the overall treatment plan.

When I accompanied Charlie to some of her initial appointments, I noticed her psychiatrist wouldn't really engage too much with me. Even if I asked questions, she would respond directly to Charlie. I guess it was early in our relationship and she probably didn't even know if I'd stick around for long enough. But over the years, we've developed a strong mutual understanding of Charlie's care and as we've progressed on this journey, the relationship and trust have continued to build.

We now have a well-established three-way communication channel where she really values my input. This helps her have a more holistic approach to Charlie's treatment and care. For example, she is aware of our goals as a couple and our plans for the future. Knowing this in advance enables us to be prepared for any potential triggers and helps her to better support us as we continue traversing life's interesting journey.

MEDICATION

I'm on a range of medications for my mental health. I take a combination of an antidepressant, mood stabiliser, and antipsychotic medication. These drugs have changed many times and the doses within those medications have also been altered and tweaked to reach an effective therapeutic dose. I also take benzodiazepines when I need them for anxiety and sleep. Each of these medications has its own benefits and side effects and it's taken a long time and a lot of trial and error to arrive at the right balance. Even now, medications are changed and altered from time to time to ensure they're working to best support me. The side effects can be mild or moderate for some, whereas for others, they can be more severe. One drug I was on caused problems with my heart and another caused a seizure which was pretty scary. It's crucial that I work with my psychiatrist and GP on any medication changes and follow their directions regarding titration of doses.

When I'm well, I take my medication as prescribed and I'm very particular about it as I know there can be serious adverse reactions if I'm not careful. I manage them myself but recently had to request my pharmacist to supply me with Webster packs after I accidentally made a medication error. A Webster pack is when the pharmacist provides your medication in a sealed packet broken down into doses per time of day. Also, when I'm relapsing and hear voices telling me not to take the medication or overdose on them, it can be extremely difficult to follow the regimen so the Webster packs are safer. That way I know exactly where I'm up to.

Having to take so many medications a day goes against the grain even when I'm well and taking them as prescribed. I struggle with having to put so many drugs into my system but I understand and accept that they help me in different ways. I worry about short and long-term effects and really wish I didn't have to take them. I feel angry with myself for needing them, so it's no wonder that I don't want to take them when I'm psychotic. However, I honestly believe I could have died without them. I was a risk to myself when I was unmedicated. I needed something to stabilise me and medication came as an integral piece of the puzzle. Now, I'm grateful for something that has given me a better life and no matter how much I fight against it, I know it's crucial.

***

Medication, whilst being a necessary part of Charlie's care, has been one of the most complex things to get right. Due to the brittle nature of the illness, Charlie needs to be on a combination of multiple medications, each having their own doses, titration scales and, of course, side effects. These need to be closely monitored and titrated. Most of the major medication changes she's had have been as an inpatient in hospital so that her body's reaction to them can be monitored and professional help is available in case of any major side effects.

I remember during one such hospital admission when her medications were being changed, Charlie had a seizure. This was understandably really terrifying for us both as Charlie had never had a seizure before. She had to be rushed to Emergency and after several tests, they concluded it was the change in medication that had caused it. So it's extremely important that any medication changes, however big or small, are done in consultation with a psychiatrist or GP where appropriate, and the correct titration plan is followed.

After a long process of trial and error involving several different medications and varying doses, we've finally landed on a medication regime that's working and can be titrated within limits when needed. However, we do understand this might need to be changed from time to time.

ELECTROCONVULSIVE THERAPY (ECT)

ECT or Electroconvulsive Therapy is a treatment where electric currents are passed through the brain to cause a mild seizure. This is done under general anaesthesia and is meant to cause stimulation in the brain to relieve symptoms. This is usually considered when other treatment options, such as medication, have been unsuccessful. I had a course of ECT about 11 years ago and it helped to dig me out of severe depression. My treatment team tried a number of medications but I was still struggling a lot. I don't remember much during this time, apart from the fact that I was an inpatient for many weeks. The ECT shifted something and I got discharged.

A couple of years ago, I was started on a course of ECT again as medication wasn't working for depression and psychosis. This time, it was far from effective, and they had to stop it when I'd had about eight out of 12 sessions. The side effects of memory loss, tearfulness, and confusion were very distressing. I also had severe back pain which my treating team didn't think was caused by the ECT, and they had to call the pain team to manage it.

Some people find ECT very helpful and I think my first course all of those years ago made a significant difference for me. However, after my recent experience, any future ECT treatments will need to be carefully considered.

***

My experience of ECT as a carer was extremely confronting. When it was suggested, I was given limited information about the treatment. We were at a crossroads not knowing what to do next. Since we knew it had helped Charlie in the past, we agreed to give it a go. All I knew was they would stimulate tiny amounts of electricity that would jolt her brain. I was told to expect that Charlie might be a bit foggy and not remember much of the procedure.

But our actual experience was much worse. Charlie's memory was severely impacted by the treatment. After each session was concluded, she couldn't remember where she was, why she was there, or what medications she was on. She couldn't even remember my phone number. I used to have to leave notes for her each day reminding her of what had happened the previous day and what the plan was for the coming day.

This loss of memory and general confusion was extremely confronting for us both. Charlie was really distressed and spent most days crying. And the severe back pain on top of this didn't help either, especially because pain is often a trigger in itself. Therefore, the treatment, in my opinion, was counterproductive.

I've since got more information on ECT, as it was suggested again at a later stage as an option. I've watched videos and read up on its effectiveness and the long-term benefits that other people have experienced. But like with all treatments, this varies for each individual, so it's best to get all the information you can before you make a decision for yourself or your loved ones.

TRANSCRANIAL MAGNETIC STIMULATION (TMS)

This treatment is also used when other treatments haven't worked. It uses magnetic fields to stimulate nerve cells in the brain to help relieve symptoms. It is non-invasive and you don't have to have it under anaesthetic. This treatment is generally used for depression, but in my case, it was used for psychosis to see if it made any difference. I had four sessions during an acute phase and unfortunately, my symptoms got worse so my psychiatrist had to stop it. I found TMS a lot less daunting than ECT. I was awake throughout and could sit in a comfortable reclining chair watching television whilst the treatment was performed.

***

TMS was described to us as tapping on the head with a hammer to stimulate certain electrodes and shift the way the brain is functioning. Its side effects were significantly less than what we experienced with ECT. The only thing Charlie experienced as a result of the treatment was a bad headache. TMS can be given to one or both sides of the brain. One session of the treatment takes about an hour all up, but the actual stimulation is for about 20 minutes.

We tried TMS at a time when Charlie was experiencing a psychotic episode and maybe the further stimulation of the brain didn't help with this. Instead, at the time what seemed to help her more was rest, complete shutdown, and some increase in medication.

Given our experience, we'd be willing to reconsider TMS at a later stage should this be suggested again as an option. But we would certainly like to discuss it in more detail next time around and perhaps explore the option of having a gap between treatments. Naturally, we would once again be guided by Charlie's treating psychiatrist and collectively make an informed decision on how and when to proceed.

***

The treatment methods covered in this chapter are specific to what is available in Australia at present. Treatments will vary depending on the diagnosis as well as where you're located.

If I had to identify one treatment that has benefitted me most, I would say it is psychotherapy. This is where I started getting the help I needed, and I would have been lost without it. However, I recognise that psychotherapy couldn't work without psychiatry and vice versa. In fact, each of the treatment methods I've had in the past or have currently couldn't work independently. It's a multi-disciplinary approach that has got me to where I am today.

CHAPTER SEVEN
SUPPORT AND STRATEGIES

Besides the treatment methods that we discussed in the previous chapter, there can also be a lot of support available through hospitals and from within the community, depending on where you're based. In some instances, your GP might be the first point of contact who can then refer you to these services. You could even contact psychotherapists or counsellors directly. There are mental health helplines and online chat forums you can reach out to, and the Emergency Department might also be available if needed.

It doesn't matter where you go for support, just as long as you start somewhere. Living with a mental health condition is frightening. You can feel isolated, scared, angry, sad, lonely, and unsure of whom to turn to. But you don't need to go through this alone. There are people out there who can help. Wherever you are and whatever your circumstances, there's somebody who can support you.

***

This is true for carers as well. I initially thought support only existed for those living with mental health conditions but I've since found out that there is help for carers too. It might not be well advertised or as easily available. Sometimes it might even be labelled differently. I myself became aware of these support networks only a couple of years ago, even though I've been a carer for much longer than that. Most often, the help, support, and resources are all out there. You can check with the treating team that works with your loved one and ask what support is available for you as their carer. This can come in various forms, both professional and personal, and we'll explore what these look like for us and what we've found to be helpful.

HOSPITAL

If we catch my symptoms early, the first step in our plan of action is to try our 'hospital at home' approach. I basically try to shut down at home and cut off all external noise to allow my brain to rest. Extra medication generally helps during these periods. This sometimes works, especially if I'm on the brink of an episode. I continue my regular sessions with my psychotherapist, and Nerissa is involved in that communication so we're all on the same page. Nerissa and I check in regularly to see where I'm at and if anything is changing. We speak to my psychiatrist as well if we need to. If this doesn't help with the voices or if they change from derogatory to commanding, I need to actually be admitted to hospital.

While I understand hospital admissions are now part of my armour and provide safety, the hospital can also be a triggering place sometimes. There have been occasions where the behaviour of other patients has left me feeling scared and vulnerable. It's also a place where I tend to feel trapped, and there have been instances in the past where I've desperately wanted to get out even though I knew I had to stay in for my own safety. Despite the pros and cons, hospital admissions have benefitted me at times when I have been a risk to myself. In such circumstances, the hospital has been the only place where I could be physically and mentally safe.

I've been a patient at both private and public hospitals and my experiences have varied each time. For me, the main benefit of a private hospital is that I can be admitted under the care of my treating psychiatrist and can communicate directly with her. In the public system, one ends up being under the care of the psychiatrist they get assigned to upon admission. While they do still consult with my psychiatrist, they are the ones in charge of everyday decisions regarding my treatment in hospital and they're also responsible for signing off on my discharge plan.

There are also other practical differences between private and public hospitals. For example, the private hospital I've been in allows patients to keep their mobile phones with them. However, in the public system, patients' phones are locked away, and they are only allowed supervised access twice a day, for an hour each. These rules are put in place to ensure patient privacy and prevent any reputational damage that might occur while they're in hospital. Patients are asked to use the hospital landline to make phone calls. Personally, I've found this really hard because hospital stays are isolating enough without being cut off from private communication with my support network. Naturally, I prefer to talk to Nerissa when I'm feeling well or when I miss her, rather than when the hospital allows me to do so.

Private hospitals have a much more structured approach towards group therapy and organise many activities where participation is strongly recommended. Some patients greatly benefit from this, but given the nature of my condition, I often find it hard to engage in group sessions when I'm severely unwell. In this regard, I prefer the approach of the public system where I can just shut down and sleep in my room and only engage with others as needed. Of course, both approaches have proved to be beneficial at various stages in my recovery.

***

One of the benefits I've come to understand with public hospitals is that admissions can occur 24/7. If the assessing doctor feels an admission is required, then the patient is admitted. If all the beds are occupied, there is the option of staying in Emergency until one becomes available in the appropriate ward. This has helped us in situations where Charlie has felt highly unsafe at home and needed to be admitted straight away. On the other hand, admissions to private hospitals are made under the recommendation of the treating psychiatrist and can only occur during business hours. So in some instances, you might have to wait a few days before you manage to secure an admission.

Irrespective of whether it's a private or a public hospital, as a carer, you can request to be involved in the care of your loved one and in decisions regarding their treatment. Of course, this is subject to the patient's consent if they are over 18 years of age. If the person being treated is happy for you as their carer to be involved in their treatment and decisions, you can request to attend appointments with their psychiatrist and treating team. On occasions where this has not been possible, I've found it beneficial to write a letter or note to the doctors outlining any concerns or questions I have regarding Charlie's care and following up with them after the appointment. I can't say that communication between me and the treating team has worked on every occasion. It's been a process of trial and error, and of course, with multiple admissions, we've learnt what works and what doesn't.

When Charlie starts feeling better, we collectively come up with a plan that supports her discharge from hospital and return home. I have found it particularly useful to be involved in this process. Often, this begins with having a few hours of leave from the hospital to better understand how she's feeling and coping outside. This then progresses to longer periods of leave and time at home. We've both found that this works really well and gives us a good understanding of how Charlie will feel once she's back home. Understandably, this varies from person to person and depends on their diagnosis and the respective hospital policy too, so it's best to discuss this with the treating team.

OUTPATIENT CRISIS TEAM

The outpatient crisis team operates within the community and responds to urgent requests from people experiencing a mental health crisis. In my experience, the team usually comprises a wide range of mental health professionals. We've often contacted this team when I've had a relapse. Nerissa has usually dealt with them as I have been very unwell on these occasions. At times, they've helped us with admissions to public hospitals. The crisis team is also involved in providing care following discharge from hospital. Usually, the team contacts me and arranges a home visit to see how I'm progressing. This has been very helpful as they have reassured us with their assessment and completed the discharge process.

***

My experience with the crisis team has been varied. I've contacted them several times when Charlie's been unwell, and each time their assessment procedure and process for hospital admission has been different. As a carer, I've found this extremely frustrating as there isn't a clear process for me to follow at a time when we're understandably really stressed, worried, and in need of help. Having to deal with professionals in the community who don't necessarily have a full view and understanding of Charlie's treatment plan has also been hard. This is one of the many reasons we decided to develop the Safety Plan.

Having this plan in place has really helped us build a more structured approach to hospital admission, where her treating team and those within the community all have access to the same plan. They now know that when I call and say Charlie needs to be in hospital, that means she needs to be admitted straight away. Ever since we've put the Safety Plan in place, we've found that the process has been much smoother for us. The crisis team professionals we've dealt with have been lovely, supportive, and willing to help, it's mainly the process itself that needs working on, so all parties concerned know what we need in a crisis.

SUPPORT WORKERS

I have support workers who assist me at home and when I'm out and about in the community. They keep me focused and committed. Having them booked in regularly helps me to get out of bed in the morning when the voices are difficult to deal with. They support me with practical chores at home and in getting out into the community for appointments and social activities. This helps to build my confidence and motivation. This is crucial for me as it enables me to stay connected with everyone around me and focus on my strengths rather than my weaknesses. It also works towards building my independence.

Prior to having this system in place, Nerissa would struggle to get me to appointments whilst juggling work commitments, which is something that became stressful for both of us. Now that we have the support to do this, it has taken the stress out of it and helped our relationship. Carers are often faced with these difficult situations so having this support has really helped both of us.

CARER SUPPORT

As a carer, it took me a long time to understand that I too needed to be cared for and that it was actually okay for me to ask for help. To be honest, at first, I wasn't even aware of what I needed or what would help me in my situation. During one of Charlie's admissions to the public hospital, an Occupational Therapist spoke with me and asked if I'd like to be referred to a carer support program. I didn't really know what this involved but out of curiosity I said, "Sure, refer me." I wasn't certain this was going to help me, but I thought there couldn't be any harm in getting referred. So I went along with the process.

That one referral changed so much for me. I was connected to a carer support program with a dedicated carer advocate. The role really does what it says, which is advocate for carers, to ensure we get the support and care we need. I reach out to my carer advocate when I need someone in my corner to help and support me. She's helped me navigate complex hospital admissions, even during the pandemic when visiting was restricted, making it easier for me to communicate with Charlie's treating team.

Through this program, I've been able to attend education and awareness sessions. These have broadened my understanding around mental health and provided me with strategies and communication tools that have not only enabled me to better care for Charlie but have also helped me prioritise self-care. I no longer feel like I'm solely responsible for everything. I'm now well-supported and have other people I can rely on who care for me while I care for Charlie.

The other thing that has really helped me is attending a carer's support group. Now, you might say, "Nope, that's not for me." Fair enough. That was my initial response too. But I was wrong. My carer support group connected me to other carers who were experiencing similar situations and had shared concerns and questions. I found a safe space where we could all learn from and leverage each other's experiences and also feel more supported as a community. Mental health can be dark and often hard to talk about in everyday life. So being part of a group where I can speak openly with people who understand what I'm going through has really helped. I no longer feel as alone because I know there are others in my situation too. We each have different journeys, but we can still help and support each other.

PRACTICAL STRATEGIES THAT HELP

One of the most important things that help me stay on track is maintaining a daily routine. This provides structure to my day. Having a fixed wake-up time, planned activities, and regular appointments helps me regulate my mind and body. I also take medications at specific times each day so the correct dosages are regularly maintained. Knowing what to expect and planning ahead helps take the stress out of my day. For example, I knew writing this book would require a lot of time and focus so setting aside time for this during the first half of the day when I have more energy and concentration was really beneficial.

Getting a good night's sleep is extremely important for me. Due to the medications I take, I need at least eight to 10 hours of sleep to function properly. I've also found that maintaining a healthy diet and getting regular exercise have a direct impact on my mental health and general well-being. A common side effect of psychiatric medication is weight gain and an increased appetite. This coupled with the lack of motivation to exercise doesn't make for a great combination. So it's vital that I maintain a healthy and balanced diet and schedule regular exercise, even if it's something simple like taking my dog out for a walk or going for a swim. This helps with my sleep routine too.

What I've also found helpful is practising mindfulness and meditation. These help keep me grounded and present in the moment and work really well as maintenance activities to increase periods of wellness. I schedule them into my routine and do them before each mealtime and before I sleep. They help me to reflect, unwind, and focus on positivity.

I also have a sensory box of items that I have collected over time that helps me cope with distressing symptoms. It includes photos of my loved ones, rugged stones, positive notes from friends and family, comforting trinkets, and textured objects. They all have a role in helping me stay connected and present. At times when I'm triggered by something at home or in hospital, my sensory box tends to help.

***

Whilst treatments and established support systems have been crucial in getting us to where we are today, our mindset also plays a huge role in moving us forward and allowing us to continue to grow through everything we face. This can be challenging at times, especially when Charlie is unwell, but we've realised that what we choose to focus on can also greatly impact our lives.

Being able to stay present and grounded in moments of high stress and anxiety has helped me navigate some extremely complex and challenging situations. I do this by focusing on the things that I can control at that moment. Even something as simple as slowing down my breathing and being more mindful of each breath has helped me regulate my own anxiety. Having routine and structure in my day and taking time out for self-care has been crucial for me. It's provided me with a level of certainty that enables me to thrive amidst situations I can't always control.

As carers, we can tend to focus on the needs of the person we're caring for and in turn neglect ourselves. There have been several occasions where I've casually put off doing something for myself, but I would never compromise on any of Charlie's needs. Over the years, I've realised how important self-care is. And actually taking time out to refill and refuel my own mind and body has in turn allowed me to be more actively present for Charlie.

A great way to do this is by having a list of self-care activities that you can do in specific blocks of time. So when things get really hectic and you're not able to spend an hour doing something you like, you know you've got a number of other things that you can do in five or 15 minutes that can help you recharge. My five-minute self-care activities include things like dancing to my favourite track, doing a short meditation, or stepping outside and breathing in some fresh air. Our lists can include anything we like doing, but what's important is that we actually use them to focus on the crucial element of self-care.

Another thing that's really helped us in our journey is practising gratitude. We started practising gratitude long before we even knew its actual benefits. After one of Charlie's initial surgeries following the accident, everything seemed to be going wrong. It felt like we had no control over how things were unfolding and in a desperate attempt to focus on something other than our present situation, we decided to write down three things that we were each grateful for. They didn't have to be big events. In fact, they were all mostly basic things, like the fact that someone had brought in a home-cooked meal for us that day. But what started out as a simple practice has now become something we constantly go back to during moments of both wellness and difficulty. Being able to find things we can be grateful for even during some of our darkest times has been paramount for us and it's something that we both practice individually, and as a couple too.

Ever since we got these support systems in place and began focusing on helpful strategies, we've both noticed changes in each other. Charlie is more independent now. There are positive shifts in her mood and she's also more aware of her own triggers and how to manage them. This has been helpful for me too as it means I'm not having to manage the stress of it all on my own. Knowing there are people we can rely on for help and being able to take time out for myself, has been hugely beneficial. It has allowed us to focus on our relationship more, support each other better, and work towards achieving our goals as individuals and as a couple. Even writing this book didn't seem like a possibility a few years ago, but now it's become a reality. And we hope our journey helps you and your loved ones in some way.

CHAPTER EIGHT
COMMUNICATION

Communication has always been at the forefront of our journey as a couple. Open and honest communication can be hard to maintain in any relationship, even without throwing PTSD and psychosis into the mix. It's been really tough for us at times, but we've continued to learn and grow over the years and we're definitely getting better at it every day.

It's no surprise that communicating with me when I'm experiencing psychosis is really difficult. This might be for a number of reasons. I might be paranoid and think that I can't trust the person talking to me. In turn, the person speaking to me may not understand this and could say or do things that aggravate the situation, even though they didn't mean to do so. I might turn inward, grow incredibly disconnected and become unable to communicate with anyone. At times like these, I am often able to send text messages or write notes to communicate my thoughts, and this has been extremely helpful for us. A text message I sent to Nerissa during one of my recent episodes is as follows:

The voices commanding me to kill myself are relentless at times and it's getting harder to cope with them. I'm scared that I'll act on them and die soon from suicide. It's such a strong feeling. I can't keep on living like this. I can't live in this fear. Every time I get on top of it I go downhill again.

Once I'm well, we talk about these messages and the fear that not only I but Nerissa naturally feels too. I can't imagine receiving a text message like this from her, so I can totally understand how terrified she must be when she reads these. During my most recent episode, she really didn't know if I'd make it through my hospital admission. So while communicating via text is invaluable, it certainly has its major stresses. For example, Nerissa has to read it alone, process it, interpret what I'm feeling, and determine what I need at that moment. All this without any further explanation from me, at least not until she receives my next response.

I also use a notebook to communicate and challenge the voices and this excerpt is quite different from the text message above:

I've spent three weeks in desperation [in hospital]. *Now left alone I fight and fight with the voices. He says 'I'm going to harm Nerissa'. He has gone for my heart. I will do anything for her. But he says I mustn't speak of this at all or there'll be consequences. This is too much pain.*

You can't touch her. She is strong. I am strong. You would be shocked at the person I have become. I will stand up and fight you. I will not follow your demands. You will not harm me or anyone I love. You are weak and pathetic.

This excerpt is an example of how we can also gain strength from our communication, no matter what form it takes. Moments like these when I'm able to stand up to the voices give us hope, hope that I'm turning a corner, hope that our future could look different. It gives us something to hang on to.

There is a lot going on inside my head when I'm psychotic so I need people to be clear and calm when they're talking to me. If someone is asking me questions, it's helpful if they can break them down into small sentences. It can be extremely hard for me to concentrate as I could be hearing highly distressing voices that are all competing for attention with the person speaking to me. Adding a loud, critical, or harsh voice to the cacophony I can already hear only escalates my distress. Thus, the approach of the other person needs to be non-threatening. During these times, I need to be spoken to quietly, and I need the other person to follow my lead in the conversation.

When speaking to someone who's going through a psychotic episode, it's important to listen and empathise with them, even if you don't understand what they're saying. Acknowledge how distressed or scared they might be feeling. Explain that you're there to support them in a non-judgmental way whilst remaining clear and calm. And respect their wishes if they don't want to talk to you. It can be really draining talking to someone when I'm psychotic, but it helps when people let me know they're around if I want to chat with them later. This is another note I left for Nerissa and a good example of when I need those around to be calm with me:

I'm feeling trapped [in the hospital]. *The front door is opening and I want to run but I know I can't. In the last hospital the doors were locked, whereas now I have the freedom if I want to take it. I'm so confused. I know my therapist explained why my abuser can't be poisoning me but I still have the same feelings. I don't want to tell Nerissa and let her down.*

Nerissa and I talk about suicide openly when I'm well and sometimes when I'm unwell too, if I'm feeling up to it. Since I can't always clearly communicate how I'm feeling, we use the 1-10 Suicide Scale to check in and determine how I'm feeling every day. If I'm sitting at an eight or above, that's a clear indication that I need to go into hospital. My therapist suggested this to help us gain better clarity on when I should go into hospital as Nerissa was being left with the huge responsibility of making this decision alone.

The other aspect of communication that's been important for us is how we communicate with our family and friends. Naturally, our approach here varies from person to person. Some people are very supportive and help Nerissa and me both individually and together. They don't always claim to understand what's going on, but they lend a listening ear and are ready to help in any way they can. These are the people we know we can rely on. Other family and friends aren't quite so involved but what's important is that we know they have our best intentions at heart and that they love us. They may just not know what to say or how best to support us with what we need. This is common with mental health as it can often be difficult to know what to say. Some people are frightened by it and think they'll say the wrong thing so they choose to stay quiet altogether. But what's helpful to me is to know they are still around if I need them, even if they don't understand all of it.

Relationships are complex and it's important to try not to judge people based on their responses. Education and awareness in this regard can help family members and friends in supporting their loved ones and that's what we try to encourage during periods of wellness so they can better support us when I'm unwell.

***

Right from the beginning, Charlie and I have always been open and honest in our communication and have always felt safe and comfortable sharing things with each other. However, when it came to discussing our experiences around mental health, some conversations were much harder than the common day-to-day conversations that most couples might have. Past relationships also impacted how safe Charlie felt about sharing her thoughts and feelings with me. Understandably, she was worried about how I'd react to all of it. Would I get angry that she was having a relapse? Would I be scared about what she was about to reveal? Would I bring up the idea of a hospital admission? Would I be able to cope with it myself?

These are all valid questions and I can understand why Charlie felt that level of hesitation. To be honest, I too didn't know how to respond to most of it. I was also worried that if I didn't respond in the appropriate way, Charlie might feel uncomfortable approaching me the next time she experiences similar thoughts.

Over the course of our relationship, there have been many moments where we both have struggled to express ourselves and respond appropriately in a given situation. We've both become better at it with time, but it's interesting to look back and see how our communication skills and strategies have evolved over the years.

For example, I am very practical and logical by nature, so the moment Charlie would share with me that the intensity of the voices was increasing or that she was experiencing relapse symptoms, I'd go straight into 'action mode' and the words I'd use to speak to her would reflect that too. So I would say things like, "Okay, given how you're feeling, here's what we should do..." and I'd just rattle off a step-by-step action plan. You see, I thought I was being helpful. I was providing useful solutions and suggesting things that I thought would help. It's how I had learnt to deal with difficult situations – identify the problem, find the solution, and implement it. Easy and simple, right?

Wrong. I soon learnt that mental health was neither easy nor simple and that it certainly couldn't be 'fixed' by a 3-step action plan. I now know that what works a lot better and is much more effective when it comes to mental health is active listening. When someone confides in us about their mental health, they're sharing something really personal that could make them feel very vulnerable. It could be something that's really hard for them to disclose or maybe even put into words. This is true in Charlie's case. And in those moments, what Charlie's often looking for is for someone to listen, to acknowledge how she's feeling, and provide reassurance. She doesn't need solutions and action plans, but simply for someone to let her know that we hear what she's saying. Over time, I've learnt and become conscious and intentional with the words I use and how I respond when Charlie shares her thoughts or feelings with me.

Nowadays, my response is more on the lines of something like this: "Thank you so much for sharing that with me. I understand that couldn't have been easy for you to do. Thank you for trusting me and feeling comfortable about letting me know. Is there anything I can do to help? Anything you feel will help you?"

Approaching the situation in this way not only reassures Charlie that I've heard and acknowledged what she's sharing with me but also creates space for her to let me know how I can help her and what she needs from me. Involving the person in making decisions about their care is very important as it helps them feel that they're in control and that you're there to help. This approach has worked wonders for us in our communication and has helped Charlie feel that she can share anything with me and know that I'll always be there for her no matter what.

Of course, this approach needs to be tweaked when it comes to suicide, suicidal ideations or potential self-harm. Below is an excerpt of a message Charlie once sent me when she was severely unwell:

"Babe I can't talk to you about this. That's really important. You mustn't say anything because he's told me I can't speak about it and I'm really scared. Please. He's telling me I must kill myself or he'll harm you. You know what he's capable of. This is a direct threat he's ordering me to do and I must keep silent"

When I read a message like this, I know immediately that she's not safe. It's too risky to stay at home. Even if I believe she won't really act on the voices, there's no way of knowing for sure. And the risk is too high. So I know at this point that she needs to go to the hospital. But she's also told me she's scared and can't talk about it. So I have to approach this in a way that makes her feel safe and reassured but also helps us arrive at the right outcome, which is getting her to agree to go into hospital. I know this isn't going to be an easy conversation but it's one that needs to happen now. I take a deep breath in and breathe out. Then I head into the room.

I sit down beside her and say, "Thank you for sending me that message. I really appreciate you sharing that with me. I know you're scared to talk, but is it okay if I talk to you about it?"

She nods as if to say okay. So I proceed. "I know you're scared right now, I imagine it's really frightening."

She nods as tears roll down her cheeks. I know she's terrified.

"It's okay," I say. "It's okay to cry. It helps release it, so cry and let it out."

She sobs and I sit with her and hold her. "I know, I understand, it's very scary isn't it?"

"Yes," she replies, and I begin to let her know that it's scary for me too. I tell her that I'm frightened and that while I know she's safe and no one is going to harm her, I can't take the risk of keeping her at home at this point. But instead of just saying, "I think you need to go to hospital," I tell her how I wouldn't be able to live with myself if something were to happen to her. I continue to explain things calmly and then approach the idea of hospital as a question.

"Do you think you'll feel safer in hospital?" I ask calmly.

She nods, which by now I know is her way of letting me know that even though she doesn't really want to go to the hospital (as most people don't), she knows it's the right thing to do, and so we proceed.

This approach works for us, but there could be cases where a person might not be able to respond, might not be able to comprehend questions, or determine the need for safety and take appropriate measures. In such cases, it's best to call the Emergency Line and get professional help. Trying various forms of communication is all well and good, but at the end of the day, safety is paramount.

Talking about suicide has become somewhat normal for us now. Not normal in the sense that we don't take it seriously and act on it appropriately, but that it's no longer a taboo or scary topic of discussion. Instead, we talk about it openly and practically now. We could be having breakfast and I might ask Charlie where she's sitting on the Suicide Scale, and whether she's having any suicidal or self-harm thoughts. Making this part of our regular conversation helps us both feel comfortable discussing the subject when things are going well and prepares us to approach it better during a rough patch.

Another thing that has really helped us is establishing different modes of communication that Charlie can use when she's unable to verbalise what's happening. We've agreed that she can text, write a note, or send an email. Charlie uses email with her psychotherapist and psychiatrist too and this has been a useful channel when she's too scared to talk. At times, even if it isn't the fear, Charlie finds it easier to express some of the harder stuff via email first, before she's able to talk it through with her therapist during the session. Establishing these different modes of communication has helped us feel more reassured, communicate better, and let each other know where we're at.

Both verbal and non-verbal communication is crucial when dealing with mental health and it's important to understand and establish the best ways you can communicate with your loved one. Above everything, approaching every situation with love and understanding, and a genuine desire to learn and support each other has really helped us both.

This approach is also useful when having conversations with others about their mental health, especially when someone says to us, "Well, actually I'm not really okay." Conversations like these can be sensitive and tricky to navigate, so below are a few things that I've found to be helpful in such instances.

The first step is to talk about mental health in the same way that we would talk about physical health, giving it equal importance, if not more. For example, we wouldn't tell someone with a broken leg to simply get up and get on with their day. So how can we expect the same thing from someone living with anxiety or depression?

There needs to be an increased level of awareness, understanding and patience when dealing with mental health. Together, we can create a safe place, a society and a community, where people know that it's okay to not be okay and where they don't feel ashamed to ask for help or admit they're struggling.

What's also important is choosing the right place and time to have a conversation. If we pick a time when we're with a big group of friends or maybe heading into a busy meeting, the person we're asking might not feel comfortable sharing how they're really feeling. Having a conversation on a one-on-one basis generally works better, but it's important to make sure that we're in a safe place where both parties feel comfortable. If the person is sitting down, it helps if we sit down as well. This way, we're at the same level as the person we're speaking with, which makes us seem more approachable and helps the other person feel comfortable sharing their feelings.

When someone tells us how they're feeling, it's important to actively listen to them. Sometimes we listen to respond rather than listening to understand. We feel compelled to say something. And when responding, we often make it about ourselves and what we think the person should do. But communication is more than just words. Sometimes, just sitting with a person, actively listening to them, letting them know they have our full attention, and simply acknowledging what they have to say can be really powerful.

As we continue this journey together, we know our communication skills and methods will keep changing and evolving. What is important for both of us is that we are committed to working on ways to better communicate with each other, our loved ones, and those in our community.

CHAPTER NINE
ACCEPTANCE

Acceptance has many facets. When you live with PTSD and schizoaffective disorder, acceptance can be a tricky thing to navigate. I have gone from fully accepting my diagnosis and complying with treatment to denying its existence altogether and then back again in a very short period of time. I have experienced sadness, anger, shock, denial, and a sense of complete numbness and lack of connectedness with everything around me. It has been a process of grief and loss. But, hope has also been a crucial part of this journey. When I'm well, I have an inherent belief that I can adjust and cope with anything that life throws at me. Now, this might be extremely challenging to access when I'm psychotic and depressed, but there's something in me that keeps me fighting. I have come back time after time. I have found ways to tell Nerissa, my psychotherapist, or my psychiatrist that I'm feeling unsafe and require additional support, and they have been able to put in place what I need each time.

Personally, grief, loss, hope, and acceptance have featured in many aspects of my life and continue to do so as part of my journey. Physically, I went from being a very active person holding down a good job to finding myself bed-bound for 11 weeks following my motorbike accident. I thought I'd been through the worst when I got discharged from the hospital and went into physical rehabilitation for the first time. But it was actually just the beginning. I had to go through a series of gruelling surgeries, ongoing rehabilitation, and even had to learn how to mobilise again. Not only have I had to cope with these physical and mental health challenges, but I have also lost out on my career and relationships, which has made acceptance so much harder.

After I was diagnosed with schizoaffective disorder and had undergone a couple of relapses, my psychiatrist mentioned that even with medication and the right treatment plans, it was likely that I'd always continue to experience residual symptoms. Which meant that the voices would never really go away completely. Acceptance and denial were battling it out in my mind. I read up on schizoaffective disorder and, somewhere, a very small part of me began to realise it was true. I continued to bargain with myself and the waves of anger and resentment came back with even greater force. Poor Nerissa had her work cut out. I was dealing with my physical injuries, adjusting to new psychiatric medication, and trying to wrangle with my mental health diagnosis. This was going to be a long process. I just couldn't bring myself to accept it.

One of the biggest hurdles that lay in the path of coming to terms with this diagnosis was accepting the need for long-term medication. With PTSD and depression, I had always believed that I would overcome them at some point. That I would get better and would no longer need to take medication. But with schizoaffective disorder, I was being told it was likely that I'd experience episodes or relapses throughout my life and would always need medication. I was left to accept that this is a brittle condition that would fluctuate over time.

I felt dejected. I was so sad. I became distant and disconnected again while I tried to process everything. What is devastating over time is that I experience this lack of acceptance and the feelings that accompany it with almost every episode of becoming unwell. Firstly, I say I don't need medication. This is often an early sign of a relapse. Nerissa and my psychotherapist are my sounding boards as I try to reason with them, I genuinely don't understand what they're saying. I spend hours reading up on schizoaffective disorder looking for a get-out clause for my diagnosis. Bargaining. I fight the same battle every time and it almost feels like going back to the beginning again. Surely they've got this wrong. The voices join in and the intensity increases. Not only do these voices tell me not to take medication, but they also say I should overdose on it. My psychotherapist reminds me of what I tell her when I'm well. That I have to take medication as prescribed or I'll become more unwell. She tells me I had asked her to remind me of this when I have other episodes. I also write it down to prompt my memory and Nerissa puts her point of view across, but even with all of this, I struggle. I feel like I've lost control of everything. I'm not in charge anymore. I want to scream and shout but I haven't got the strength or ability to do it. It's as if no one understands me. I feel so alone in the depths of despair and there's no way out. I have all this support around me yet I can't connect with anyone.

When I had my amputation, acceptance was quite different. I felt a huge sense of relief. I had battled for four years with pain. I had to learn to use a wheelchair and live with massively restricted mobility. I had gone through endless surgeries only to find that they were unsuccessful. So I didn't struggle to accept my new amputee status and actually embraced it. As I went through rehabilitation and started learning to walk again, I felt positive I had made the right decision. I was truly able to accept it, which felt very different to my experiences with my mental health. In fact, Nerissa struggled to accept it more than I did. She felt the decision to have an amputation was fast, whereas I'd actually been adjusting to the possibility for a long time. Of course, I went through highs and lows. The first time I tried my prosthetic on to walk, I stood at the parallel bars and was stuck. I was trying to get my brain to connect with my leg, but nothing happened. I felt disheartened and frustrated but I could accept that this was okay, it was part of the process. However, when it comes to my mental health, I can be paranoid, delusional, and irrational. There often isn't any room for reasoning.

There is one area, however, in which my leg causes challenges for my mental health. I often believe there is a chip in my leg that, since my accident, has been transmitting and broadcasting my thoughts to those around me. This thought isn't always there; it would recur most prominently after I'd had surgery and believed that it had been planted there during the procedure. However, I continue to experience this now despite not having had surgery for a while.

The interrelated complexities around my mental and physical health have also had an impact on my career. I was an RN before my accident and couldn't return to those duties due to my physical limitations. So I tried a number of desk jobs, but these triggered my anxiety and led to a series of psychotic episodes, resulting in hospital admissions and serious ill-health. This was when we decided that I had to accept that I couldn't work unless I had long periods in remission. Besides losing my physical health, I was now also losing my career, which I had to accept. This was a big adjustment but it resulted in some improvement in my mental health, despite ongoing episodes.

Relationships are also a challenge when you're living with a mental health condition and that's one of the hardest things to accept. Nerissa and I have been on a rollercoaster since we met.

Thankfully, we've become more skilled at dealing with it as time has passed but there are still some areas around my mental health that feel like Groundhog Day. When I'm well, we plan for the future, have fun and laugh together, and feel so connected. We love each other and feel deep gratitude for what we have. Yet it can all change in an instant, sometimes with no warning or obvious trigger. Our love never fails but I'm 'absent' during these periods and Nerissa never really knows when I'm going to be back fully.

While I've identified the difficulties we face living with acceptance in our lives, that's exactly what we're doing; accepting it and living it. The diagnosis takes time away from us. It can curb our enjoyment in life. It challenges our relationship. I can't always accept my condition when I'm unwell. But this isn't who we are. This is only a very small part of us, and we're not just surviving, but we're smashing it!

***

Acceptance is an interesting word and it can often mean different things at different stages of our journey.

When we think of acceptance, we may at times associate it with hopelessness. We may think that if we accept where we're at today, then that means we've given up, and we can't get to where we want to be. Sometimes, we tend to see acceptance as stagnation, without hope or possibility of moving forward.

But I'd like to encourage you to shift your perspective on acceptance. The way I see it, acceptance is an understanding and awareness of where we are today, of our current situation, which then allows us to move forward and grow through to where we need to be.

Think of it as using a navigation system. In order to get to where you want to be, you need to first know where you're at — your current location. You need to then enter your current location, point A, into the navigation system to be able to get to your destination, point B. Similarly, acceptance, for me, began when I was able to fully acknowledge and understand what was really involved in caring for someone living with a chronic mental health condition — the good, bad and often very raw. All of it.

Initially, I naively thought I could fix things. I thought that if I did everything I possibly could, if we followed all the medication and treatment plans, if I knew all of Charlie's triggers, then I could fix this. I could prevent her from having a relapse and I could, potentially, get rid of the condition. Then when she got unwell, I felt terrible. I felt like I had let her down, like I had let myself down, and I really blamed myself for it. I thought, well I've done everything I can possibly do, and yet we're back here again. I really believed that if I had known more, done more, and been there more, then maybe Charlie wouldn't have relapsed.

But over the years, I've realised that it's out of my control. I can't cure the illness and I can't prevent a relapse. So I've learnt to step back and allow it to run its course. Journeying through many such cycles has allowed us to build resilience. We now know that even when things get really tough, Charlie will turn a corner and we will come through. And this acceptance has allowed us to grow through our experiences and take learnings from each one into the next.

When Charlie goes through a severe period of being unwell, she often doesn't remember a lot of what's happened. But for me, those experiences and feelings are still raw. I remember every tiny little detail and incident. So the trauma for me is still very real, even after Charlie's no longer experiencing it. And battling those emotions has often been extremely challenging.

I think the realisation hit me a few years ago when Charlie had been in and out of the hospital in quick succession, often having to remain in for several weeks at a time. It hit me then, that this was going to be a marathon, not a sprint, and if we were going to survive this – if our relationship was going to survive this – then we would have to come to terms with some harsh realities. I would have to adjust and reset some of my expectations, not only as an individual, but also our expectations as a couple – for our relationship, and for our future.

As a carer, I feel acceptance for me spans across different levels. There's acceptance of the illness itself, acceptance of what it means for our relationship, acceptance of my own limitations as a carer and acceptance around what it means for our future. I don't believe I came to a state of acceptance for all of this at once. It's been more of a gradual process over the years for me, and I'm still learning and growing.

The first bit of acceptance for me was around the illness itself. It was understanding and being able to accept the fact that I can't cure it and I can't stop relapses from happening. To think I could do any of that would only be setting myself and our relationship up for failure. Of course, there are a number of things we can do to increase the periods of wellness and improve how we live with it so it doesn't take over our lives. Acceptance for me has also been in the realisation that Charlie's mental health diagnosis is the same as any physical ailment. A person living with a mental health condition is no different from someone living with cancer or a chronic physical health condition, and if we treat both the same, then there's no difference in the acceptance either.

When it comes to acceptance with regard to our relationship, what's really helped me is being able to separate Charlie from the illness. Now you might say that's not possible because she comes with it, but let me explain what I mean by this. What's helped me is to not hold the symptoms and behaviours associated with the diagnosis against Charlie. It isn't her fault that these are the symptoms of the condition. When you can see your loved one as separate from the illness, and not let it define them and your relationship, that goes a long way in reaching a level of acceptance.

For example, when Charlie is severely unwell, she can often shut down, and not want to communicate or interact much. She can also get irritable and snappy, and stay in bed for extended periods of time. Initially, I would get upset as this impacted our relationship as a couple. It impacted how we communicated and also the amount of quality time we got to spend with each other, and I'd find myself getting irritated too in response. Over the years though, I've realised that this is definitely not because Charlie doesn't want to spend time with me or is choosing to be irritable. It's the intensity of the voices, the hallucinations and delusions that are preventing her from being able to be present with me. If she could, I know and believe that it's not how she'd choose to respond.

When it comes to my role as a carer, it took me even longer to gain full acceptance of what this actually meant. You see, as carers, we can often put a lot of pressure on ourselves. Pressure to know the answers, pressure to get everything right all the time. On top of that, there is the added pressure of needing to be there, to show up, and to know what to do and say to best support our loved ones. But in all fairness, we as carers are learning too. Most of the time we come into this cold, like in my instance, where I knew nothing about the condition, what was helpful, or how to help. I was learning, discovering, figuring things out at the same time as Charlie.

So in this regard, acceptance for me was around acknowledging the fact that I am a carer and will continue to be, but with that also came the awareness that I couldn't do it on my own. I learnt that if I did, in fact, want to continue the marathon, if we wanted to thrive and not just survive, then I'd need help. Help in understanding more about the condition, help with better strategies that I can use for myself as well as with Charlie, and also help with how I myself coped with all of it. Being able to ask for help really turned things around for us and we know that we'll continue needing help as we keep learning and growing.

In terms of what our future holds, I am truly in a place of acceptance. I know that this mental health condition will continue to exist, it's going to be a part of our lives, but it's not our whole lives. And our whole life doesn't have to revolve around this. This realisation has allowed us to switch our focus from 'I' to 'we', and to reach out and ask for help. In doing so, we've been able to shift our focus from illness to wellness. We know this isn't miraculously going to go away, but over the years we've learnt not just to live with it but to build a life around it, one that doesn't break down or fall apart even when things do go wrong, as we know they will. There will be relapses, there will be further hospital admissions, there will absolutely be things that we will both learn about ourselves and our relationship. But that's exactly it. With acceptance, it's a journey, not a final destination.

Point B keeps moving, just as point A does.

CHAPTER TEN
HOPE

Writing this book has been a really cathartic experience. Through this, we've both learnt a great deal about ourselves, about each other, and about our journey together as a couple. We hope our shared perspectives have helped provide you with insight and awareness on navigating life with a mental health diagnosis.

Our journey together has been a crazy rollercoaster ride of many highs and lows. Whether you're trying to manage your own condition or care for someone else, dealing with a mental health diagnosis is challenging for everyone involved. It's never really a one-person diagnosis. And it often has a ripple effect on the various people in our lives, be it friends, family, our community, or the healthcare professionals involved.

However, for us, the good patches have certainly outweighed the difficult times and there have been definite wins along the way. We believe our relationship is richer for having been on this journey as it's taught us so much and brought us closer together. We feel extremely grateful to have been able to learn from all that has been thrown our way, and we continue to hold on to that faith and gratitude as we navigate life and look forward to the future.

Below are a few key things that have really helped us grow through our mental health journey together, and we hope that these will help you too:

Know your limits: Know that the experiences of a carer might be very different to that of the person being cared for. Each of you might have your own fears, concerns, triggers and anxiety, and that's understandable. Each of you might need to process loss and grief differently. The range of mixed emotions you experience can be significantly different from what your loved one might be experiencing. So allow yourself to process those emotions and know that it's okay to feel the way you do. For the person who's living with the diagnosis, it can often take time for them to accept their condition and adjust to living life with it. For the carer, it can take a while to come to terms with their role and responsibilities.

As you interact with people living with mental health conditions as well as their carers, know that while their experiences might be similar to yours, their circumstances could be vastly different. So try not to compare your journeys but instead, where possible, learn what's working for others and consider whether you might be able to implement something similar that works for you. Be kind to yourself, celebrate the wins, even (and especially) the small ones, and allow yourself to grow through the process.

Ask for help: Some days it can feel like you're carrying the weight of the world on your shoulders. The strain and responsibility you feel can wear you down. And in those moments, it might be difficult to figure out what you need that can help you. You may think that trying to work it out on your own will be easier than asking for help or trying to articulate your needs. We understand that, we've both felt it too. But you don't have to go it all alone. Even when you don't know what you might need, there are people who can help you figure it out.

It takes courage to ask for help. And we both know it's not easy to admit that you need help. But we can honestly tell you that in doing so, you will feel a lot more empowered and better able to engage with your loved ones.

Build a support network around you: This can be personal and professional. We've both found it invaluable to have a multi-disciplinary team of treating professionals assist us along our journey. But it's only in recent years that we've understood the benefits of having a strong personal support network that includes our friends, family, and people in the community. These are people who you can lean on and who can support you through the rough patches so you don't have to juggle everything on your own.

Open and honest communication: For us, this has been at the core of it all. In today's world, there are so many different ways that we can communicate and we've shared how various forms of communication continue to help us every day. Communication is a two-way process, and listening is almost always more important than actually saying something. It's really important to establish multiple channels of communication and figure out which are the best ways for you to connect with your loved one. Find what works for you both, and work on them during periods of wellness, so they are strongly established when you need to rely on them in times of high stress and crisis.

Focus on wellness: This can be hard given the cyclic nature of mental health as relapses can be relentless at times. But doing this consistently has been a real game-changer and shifted things drastically for us. During periods of wellness, it's really important to spend quality time with your loved ones. Make the most of these times by doing things that refuel you and refill your cup. Make good memories that will sustain you and that you can look back on when times get tough. Focusing on the 'wellness' rather than the 'illness' is what helps us to keep growing through our experiences and gives us continued hope for our future.

Even if it is a different reality, sharing our stories and talking about mental health helps break the stigma and normalise the conversation. Our experiences might be varied and our journeys may be different. But if each of us start tuning in to the mental health and well-being of ourselves, our loved ones, and that of the wider community, together, we can help create a more inclusive and accepting world.

Finally, know that it's okay to not be okay. Whatever your situation, whatever you're dealing with, there is help available and there is always someone you can reach out to for support. You are not alone. So please, ask for help. And know that this too will pass and things will get better. You will turn a corner and there will be a way forward. There is always hope.

APPENDIX

Mental Health Safety Plan including the Voices and Suicide Rating Scale

Patient's Full Name	Preferred Name	Date of Birth
Psychiatrist's Name	Contact Details	Appointment Frequency
Psychotherapist's Name	Contact Details	Appointment Frequency
General Practitioner's Name	Contact Details	Appointment Frequency
Case Manager's Name	Contact Details	Appointment Frequency

Medications (as at): DD/MM/YY

When (Timing)	What (Name of Medication)	How much (Dosage)
Morning		
Afternoon		
Evening		
Night		
As Required		

Allergic reactions to medications	Describe the reactions
Triggers and warning signs	**Strategies that help**
Symptoms	**Episodes**

Helpful information to know in a crisis

Voices and Suicide Rating Scale

Voices: 0 = good, 10 = bad
Baseline for voices: __/10

Suicide: 0 = good, 10 = bad
Baseline for suicide: __/10

Score	How I'm feeling	What I Need
0/10		
1/10		
2/10		
3/10		
4/10		
5/10		
6/10		
7/10		
8/10		
9/10		
10/10		

This is the scale that works for us, however it can be adapted to suit your needs or that of your loved one. It's best to work with your treating team to ensure it is integrated into your treatment plan and everyone is on the same page.

Notes

Made in the USA
Monee, IL
04 November 2026

67383628R00056